THE ADHD ADVANTAGE

Why Different Brains Thrive

in A Distracted World

SHAWN TAYLOR

Table of Contents

CHAPTER ONE

Introduction

Welcome to "The ADHD Advantage: Why Different Brains Thrive in a Distracted World." ADHD sufferers have a unique set of cognitive traits that help them cope with constant distractions and growing attention demands.

ADHD is characterized by inattention, impulsivity, and hyperactivity. This book challenges the narrative by exploring ADHD's untapped potential and inherent advantages. It seeks to reframe ADHD from a deficit to a diverse and valuable neurological variation.

We'll cover ADHD's definition, symptoms, and diagnosis here. We will dispel ADHD myths and explain this neurodevelopmental condition.

This book discusses ADHD brain strengths and perspectives. Neurodiversity and celebrating cognitive differences will be discussed. Understanding ADHD cognitive traits helps us harness their power and advantage in various areas of life.

We will discuss how ADHDers can use their academic, professional, and social challenges to succeed. We empower ADHDers to succeed in life by helping them manage symptoms, develop executive functioning skills, and create a supportive environment.

We will also discuss how ADHDers can succeed in a distracted world. We will offer practical advice to improve focus, productivity, and creativity in an age of constant technological distractions.

This book features inspiring ADHD role models who overcame obstacles and used their unique cognitive strengths to achieve greatness. These stories remind us that ADHD is an inspiration and motivator, not a handicap.

We will provide a comprehensive list of resources, including professional help, support groups, and recommended reading materials, to help ADHD patients discover, grow, and fulfill.

"The ADHD Advantage: Why Different Brains Thrive in a Distracted World" invites you on a transformative exploration of ADHD, offering new perspectives, practical strategies, and empowering insights. This book will help you understand and support ADHD, whether you have it or not. Let's start this enlightening journey.

CHAPTER TWO

Understanding ADHD

What is ADHD?

Attention Deficit Hyperactivity Disorder (ADHD) is a neurodevelopmental disorder that manifests in varying degrees across the lifespan. It's characterized by inattention, hyperactivity, and impulsivity that last for extended periods of time and get in the way of daily life and general well-being. Genes, brain anatomy and function, and environmental factors all play a role in the development of attention deficit hyperactivity disorder (ADHD).

ADHD Symptoms and Diagnosis

Individuals with ADHD may experience a wide range of symptoms, but most fall into two broad categories: inattention and hyperactivity/impulsivity. Symptoms of inattention include struggling to maintain focus, forgetfulness, disorganization, and a propensity to get sidetracked easily. Fidgeting, talking too much, not waiting one's turn, and making hasty decisions are all symptoms of hyperactivity and impulsivity.

ADHD can only be diagnosed after a thorough evaluation by medical experts like psychiatrists and psychologists. They evaluate symptoms and rule out other potential causes using the standardized criteria outlined in diagnostic manuals like the Diagnostic and Statistical Manual of Mental Disorders (DSM-5). Typically, the evaluator will speak with the subject, distribute questionnaires, and watch how they act in various contexts.

Myths and Misconceptions about ADHD

Many people have false beliefs about ADHD, which can lead to discrimination and misunderstanding. Some prevalent misconceptions include:

ADHD is not a real disorder: Extensive scientific research has established ADHD as a genuine and diagnosable neurodevelopmental disorder. It's not just a matter of not trying or being undisciplined.

ADHD only affects children: ADHD is typically identified in young people, but its symptoms may continue into later life. Many people are diagnosed when the condition has progressed significantly.

ADHD is caused by bad parenting or a lack of discipline: In addition to its strong hereditary component, ADHD is a neurobiological disorder. No amount of strictness or lack thereof can be blamed.

Medication is the only treatment option: Medication is an important part of treating ADHD, but it is not the only option. Therapy, behavioral strategies, and changes in lifestyle can all be helpful in reducing symptoms and increasing functionality.

People with ADHD are unintelligent or lazy: Individuals with ADHD can excel in a variety of fields with the right amount of support and accommodations, proving that the disorder does not correlate with lower IQ. Problems with attention regulation and executive functioning are at the root of ADHD, not a lack of intelligence or effort.

By debunking these false beliefs, we can help others develop a more nuanced and compassionate understanding of ADHD and work together to create a welcoming community for those living with the disorder.

CHAPTER THREE

The ADHD Brain: Unique Perspectives and Strengths

In this chapter, we'll look at the specific mental characteristics of ADHD and highlight the unique insights and strengths that people with the disorder often bring to the table. Inclusion and creativity can flourish in a society where the special qualities of the ADHD brain are recognized and celebrated.

Neurodiversity: Embracing Differences

ADHD and other neurological differences are viewed as variations of the human brain by proponents of the neurodiversity theory, rather than as deficits or disorders. It questions the concept of a "normal" or "typical" brain and encourages people to see the value in differences in how their brains work.

Adopting a neurodiverse outlook means shifting from viewing ADHD as a deficit to appreciating it as a distinctive way of perceiving and responding to the world. It advocates for communities that welcome and appreciate the unique contributions of people with ADHD.

Adopting a neurodiverse mindset acknowledges that people with ADHD have distinct ways of thinking and solving problems, as well as developing new ideas. These varying points of view have the potential to stimulate creative and original thought, which in turn may lead to novel discoveries and ground-breaking developments.

Cognitive Traits Associated with ADHD

The ADHD mind is characterized by a unique set of cognitive traits that, while problematic in some contexts, can be highly advantageous in others. ADHD is often accompanied by the following cognitive characteristics:

Divergent Thinking: People with ADHD are known to be highly inventive and creative. Their ability to see patterns where there are none and to think creatively can yield original ideas and fresh viewpoints.

Hyperfocus a state of intense concentration and absorption in a task of interest, can occur in people with ADHD, even though they may have trouble maintaining attention in some situations.

Individuals with ADHD are capable of extraordinary productivity and engrossing engagement during periods of hyperfocus.

Rapid Information Processing: Research has shown that people with ADHD have faster cognitive processing speeds. Rapid pattern recognition, rapid connection making, and rapid response time are all made possible by this high processing speed.

Multitasking: Research suggests that people with ADHD, contrary to popular belief, can multitask effectively when involved in activities that are in line with their interests or stimulate their brains. In some situations, being able to process multiple data streams at once can be helpful.

Outside-the-Box Thinking: Individuals with ADHD often demonstrate a unique and non-linear thinking style. They have the ability to think outside the box, which often leads to novel insights and novel approaches to old problems.

Harnessing the Power of ADHD

The key to unlocking the full potential of attention deficit hyperactivity disorder (ADHD) is capitalizing on the unique cognitive traits and strengths associated with the condition. Here are some ways to put ADHD to good use:

Capitalizing on Hyperfocus: Identify and foster hyperfocus by designing activities around one's passions and providing a stimulating setting. Individuals with ADHD can be highly productive and successful by making use of their heightened capacity for focused attention.

Embracing Flexibility: In both your personal and professional life, stress the importance of being pliable and adaptable. People with ADHD tend to flourish in fluid settings that encourage experimentation and novelty.

Leveraging Creativity: Involve people with ADHD in activities that allow them to express themselves creatively and make use of their unique ability to think outside the box. Expressing and channeling one's creative energies can be accomplished through the practice of art, music, writing, or entrepreneurship.

Building Support Systems: Create a solid network of people who care and who are familiar with the advantages and disadvantages of living with ADHD. Experts in the medical field, counseling services, life coaching, or community support groups may all fit into this category.

Utilizing Technology and Tools: Employ modern organizational and productivity aids to get more done in less time. Those who suffer from attention deficit hyperactivity disorder (ADHD) can benefit from the use of digital tools such as calendars, reminders, note-taking apps, and organizational software.

Recognizing and embracing ADHD can help people reach their full potential, which in turn boosts their sense of accomplishment, happiness, and self-worth. Individuals with ADHD can bring unique insights to society and help make the world a better, more progressive place for everyone.

CHAPTER FOUR

Challenges Faced by Individuals with ADHD

Academic and Professional Challenges

The academic and occupational environments can be particularly difficult for people with ADHD. Problems with planning ahead, starting new tasks, staying focused, and finishing old ones are all examples of this. ADHD's impairments in executive functioning can get in the way of one's ability to succeed in school and the workplace.

Students with ADHD may have trouble paying attention in class, remembering what they've learned, and prioritizing their work. They may have trouble paying attention to detail, keeping track of their resources, and completing tasks by the due date. Academic performance may suffer, stress levels may rise, and frustration may increase as a result of these obstacles.

Workplace productivity, deadline adherence, and organizational skills are all areas where people with ADHD may struggle. They may have trouble organizing their time, setting priorities, and juggling multiple commitments. Work productivity, relationships with coworkers, and opportunities for professional growth may all suffer as a result of these challenges.

Individuals with ADHD face unique challenges in school and the workplace, but with the right support, accommodations, and strategies, they can achieve great things. Individuals with ADHD can succeed in these settings by implementing strategies such as task simplification, the use of visual aids and reminders, and the establishment of routines.

Social and Emotional Challenges

The social and emotional well-being of a person with ADHD can be negatively affected by the symptoms they experience. Individuals with ADHD often face the following social and emotional difficulties::

Impulsivity and Social Interactions: Interrupting others, talking when it's not your turn, and other impulsive behaviors can be problematic in social settings. This can put a strain on relationships and make people feel rejected or alone.

Emotional Regulation: Those who suffer from Attention Deficit Hyperactivity Disorder (ADHD) may struggle to control their feelings, which can manifest as mood swings, irritability, or outbursts. Relationships suffer, frustration and low self-esteem are fostered, and all because of emotional dysregulation.

Social Perception and Communication: The inability to read social cues, comprehend nonverbal communication, or accurately gauge the emotional state or motivations of others may be exacerbated in people with ADHD. This can make it hard to make friends and keep them, as well as lead to misunderstandings.

Self-Esteem and Self-Concept: A person's sense of self and confidence can take a hit when they're confronted with adversity in their academic or professional life or in their personal relationships. Feelings of inadequacy and self-doubt can develop after repeatedly encountering obstacles or receiving criticism.

To successfully navigate social interactions and cultivate positive relationships, people with ADHD must first develop strong social and emotional skills. Improving one's social and emotional health can be accomplished through efforts such as studying and practicing social skills, consulting a therapist or counselor, learning to control one's emotions, and surrounding oneself with caring people.

ADHD and Mental Health

Individuals with ADHD often also struggle with the co-occurrence of another mental health disorder. Substance use disorders, anxiety disorders, depression, ODD, and conduct problems frequently occur together.

The presence of these co-occurring disorders has been shown to worsen ADHD symptoms and reduce both functioning and quality of life. Anxiety and depression, for instance, have been shown to disrupt focus, motivation, and efficiency in the workplace and the classroom. Substance abuse disorders may develop when people with ADHD resort to self-medication or unhealthy coping mechanisms.

It is essential to diagnose and treat ADHD alongside any comorbid mental health conditions. Medication, therapy (like cognitive-behavioral therapy), and behavioral and nutritional changes may all be part of an integrative treatment plan. Improvements in functioning, well-being, and coping with the difficulties of ADHD can result from the early identification and treatment of mental health issues.

The success, happiness, and overall quality of life of people with ADHD can be improved by recognizing and addressing the challenges they face in academic, professional, social, and emotional domains, and then providing the necessary support and creating environments that do just that.

CHAPTER FIVE

The ADHD Advantage

Rethinking ADHD: Shifting Perspectives

It is crucial to question established assumptions and reevaluate our current understanding of ADHD if we are to fully understand and value the ADHD advantage. ADHD is often portrayed in a negative light, but by changing our perspective, we can see the gifts and talents that those with the disorder bring to the world.

Understanding the unique ways that people with ADHD think, process information, and approach challenges can be facilitated by recasting ADHD as a neurological variation rather than a disorder. With this new lens, we can focus less on the weaknesses of the ADHD brain and more on its incredible potential.

Embracing Neurodiversity in the Modern World

Recognizing the value of the special contributions made by people with ADHD requires a society that embraces neurodiversity. ADHD is not a flaw that needs fixing; rather, it is a normal variation of the human brain, and neurodiversity encourages us to see it as such. It questions the validity of a universal solution and highlights the value of recognizing and appreciating individual differences in how we think.

Accepting people with different neurological make-ups is more important than ever in today's fast-paced, competitive world. When it comes to solving problems, making decisions, and being creative, the ADHD mind offers a new and interesting perspective. Inclusion and creativity can flourish when people from all walks of life are encouraged to bring their unique perspectives to the table.

Unleashing the Potential of ADHD

The key to unlocking the potential of attention deficit hyperactivity disorder (ADHD) is capitalizing on the advantages of the disorder. Key approaches to unlocking the full potential of ADHD include:

Identifying and Cultivating Strengths: It is crucial to appreciate and capitalize on the gifts of people with ADHD. Skills like creativity, divergent thinking, out-of-the-box problem solving, and laser-like focus could fall into this category. Individuals with ADHD can achieve success in a variety of settings by zeroing in on and honing their existing strengths.

Developing Executive Functioning Skills: Individuals with ADHD often struggle with executive functioning skills like organization, time management, planning, and self-regulation. Individuals can improve their ability to manage their academic, professional, and personal lives by participating in carefully designed interventions like cognitive-behavioral therapy or executive functioning coaching.

Providing Accommodations and Support: It's crucial to create a setting that works for people with ADHD and their specific requirements. Methods for accomplishing this goal include the use of visual aids, the introduction of systematic approaches, the provision of adaptable working or learning environments, and the delivery of clear and concise instructions. Individuals with ADHD can flourish and perform to their full potential with the help of accommodations and support.

Fostering a Positive Mindset: People with ADHD benefit greatly from being exposed to a positive outlook. Challenges can be reframed as learning experiences, successes can be celebrated, and self-acceptance can be encouraged. Individuals can overcome challenges, increase self-assurance, and appreciate their own strengths by practicing resilience and adopting a growth mindset.

Seeking Personalized Strategies and Support: Treatments that help one person with ADHD might not benefit another. Seek out methods of intervention and assistance that are tailored to your unique set of skills, obstacles, and aspirations. In order to gain insight, guidance, and encouragement, it may be helpful to consult with healthcare professionals, therapists, coaches, or join support groups.

When people with ADHD are able to tap into their full potential, they not only improve their own lives but also make invaluable contributions to the world at large. Individuals with ADHD have an advantage because of their unique perspectives, creative thinking, and other skills. A more welcoming, inventive, and prosperous world is the result of a society that recognizes and celebrates the ADHD advantage.

CHAPTER SIX

Strategies for Success

Managing ADHD Symptoms

Those who suffer from attention deficit hyperactivity disorder (ADHD) can greatly benefit from learning to control their symptoms. Methods that have proven useful in the control of ADHD symptoms include:

Medication: If you think medication might help with your ADHD symptoms, talk to your doctor about your options. Medication can help many people with ADHD with focus, attention, and impulse control.

Therapy: Cognitive-behavioral therapy (CBT) is one form of therapy that can help people with ADHD learn effective coping strategies. Organization, time management, emotion regulation, and problem solving are all skills that can be improved through therapy.

Structured Routines and Schedules: Setting up regular routines and schedules can give people with ADHD a sense of stability and predictability, which can aid in their ability to stay on task. Tasks can be completed more efficiently if they are broken down into smaller, more manageable steps and firm deadlines are established.

Time Management Techniques: To better manage one's time, it can be helpful to employ time management strategies like prioritization, reminders, and the use of timers or alarms. Making use of a planner app or calendar can also help you keep your life in order.

Environmental Modifications: Individuals with ADHD are more likely to be productive in a low-distraction setting. Assigning a distraction-free space to work or study in, investing in noise-cancelling headphones, clearing the desk of unnecessary items, and restricting access to electronics like smartphones and social media are all good examples.

Developing Executive Functioning Skills

Improving one's ability to plan, organize, and carry out tasks is known as executive functioning, and it is crucial for people with ADHD. Ways to hone your executive-level brainpower are detailed below.:

Break Tasks Down: Tasks can seem less daunting if you divide them into smaller, more manageable chunks. Individuals with ADHD can benefit from this method because it encourages a methodical, step-by-step approach to problem solving.

Utilize Visual Aids: Organization and planning can be facilitated by visual aids like checklists, calendars, and color-coded systems. They aid people with ADHD in keeping track of due dates, top priorities, and other tasks by providing visual cues.

Practice Self-Monitoring: One way to avoid getting sidetracked is to train oneself to be more self-aware and self-monitoring. Keeping tabs on oneself and making necessary adjustments on a regular basis can do wonders for concentration and output.

Improve Time Estimation: People with ADHD frequently under-estimate the amount of time necessary to complete tasks. Time management can be improved through practice, specifically through learning to estimate time and allocate it appropriately.

Seek Professional Support: Executive function can be improved with the help of a coach or therapist who specializes in working with people who have attention deficit hyperactivity disorder (ADHD). These experts can be invaluable in assisting with strategy development and providing accountability and support.

Building a Supportive Environment

Creating a supportive environment is crucial for individuals with ADHD to thrive and succeed. Here are strategies for building a supportive environment:

Communicate Needs: It's important to be honest about your situation with those closest to you, such as family, friends, teachers, and coworkers. If you tell people about your experiences with ADHD, they will be better able to help you.

Establish Clear Expectations: Individuals with ADHD benefit from a clear set of expectations at home, school, and the workplace to eliminate ambiguity and miscommunication. Having a set of rules and expectations in place gives people a sense of direction and helps them zero in on doing their best to meet those requirements.

Advocate for Accommodations: If necessary, look for places of study or employment that can accommodate your special needs. Extra time on tests and homework, better seating arrangements, and use of specialized equipment are all examples of reasonable accommodations.

Surround Yourself with Supportive Individuals: Create a group of people who will always have your back and who know and appreciate you for who you are, flaws and all. You can find comfort, encouragement, and useful advice from people like family, friends, mentors, and support groups.

Practice Self-Care: Get regular exercise, a good night's sleep, nutritious food, and a handle on your stress levels. Taking care of one's mental and physical health aids in concentration, stamina, and general effectiveness.

Successful and satisfying lives can be achieved by people with ADHD if they learn to control their symptoms, improve their executive functioning, and surround themselves with positive people. Keep in mind that your best approach may differ from someone else's, so it's important to try out different things and get help from experts as necessary.

CHAPTER SEVEN

Thriving in a Distracted World

Navigating Technology and Distractions

People with attention deficit hyperactivity disorder (ADHD) have it particularly tough in today's highly distractible digital environment. Here are some methods for dealing with gadgets and other sources of distraction:

Mindful Technology Use: Think about how much time and effort you put into using technology. Limit your access to technology by scheduling time each week when you won't be using any gadgets. Make use of browser add-ons or productivity software that restricts your ability to use certain websites or programs while you're trying to focus on work or school.

Create a Distraction-Free Environment: Choose an area free of distractions to work in. Finding a quiet place, putting on noise-cancelling headphones, and putting away potential distractions like phones and notifications are all good ways to achieve this.

Time Chunking: Tasks will seem less overwhelming if you divide them up and give yourself dedicated work periods. If you're having trouble staying on task and keeping your focus, try using a timer or the Pomodoro Technique (working for a set time period, then taking short breaks).

Practice Attention-Regulating Techniques:
If you're having trouble staying on task and ignoring distractions, try some attention-regulating techniques like meditation or deep breathing. Through repeated practice, these methods teach the brain to shift focus and increase self-regulation.

Cultivating Focus and Productivity

Cultivating focus and productivity is essential for thriving in a distracted world. Here are strategies to enhance focus and productivity:

Prioritize and Plan: Sort your to-dos in order of importance and urgency, and make a detailed plan. In order to keep going and avoid getting overwhelmed, it can be helpful to break down larger tasks into smaller, more manageable steps.

Utilize External Supports: People with ADHD can benefit from using external supports such as visual aids, reminders, and organizational tools to help them maintain a consistent routine and maintain their focus. Keep track of important dates, meetings, and tasks with the help of a calendar, a task management app, or a traditional paper planner.

Minimize Multitasking: While it may seem productive to juggle multiple tasks at once, people with ADHD may actually be less effective when doing so. Keep your mind on just one thing at a time to avoid distractions and produce better results.

Utilize Strengths and Interests: Capitalize on what you enjoy doing to boost concentration and interest. Include things that interest you or have meaning to the task at hand to increase your enjoyment of it.

Enhancing Creativity and Innovation

People with ADHD are known to have exceptional creative and innovative skills. Methods to promote original thought include the following:

Embrace Divergent Thinking: Divergent thinking, in which many ideas are generated and unconventional solutions are considered, is a strength of many people with ADHD. Take pride in your ability to question established norms and think independently.

Create a Stimulating Environment: Fill your environment with creative catalysts like books, art, and music. Try working in a coffee shop, or spending time in nature, to see which setting inspires you the most.

Allow for Flexibility and Variety: Incorporate pliability into your processes and plans. People with ADHD do best in settings that offer plenty of opportunities to switch things up. To keep things from getting boring, take breaks, switch up your routine, or try something new.

Collaborate and Seek Different Perspectives: Take part in group efforts or try to see things from other people's points of view. Individuals with ADHD can gain from the perspectives and advice of others, which can help to stimulate thought and open up new avenues for expression.

People with ADHD can succeed in today's multitasking society by learning to manage their time effectively, avoiding distractions, and improving their concentration, productivity, and originality. To fully realize one's potential, it is necessary to strike a balance between capitalizing on the advantages presented by ADHD and coping with the difficulties caused by distractions.

CHAPTER EIGHT

Success Stories and Role Models

Real-Life Examples of Successful Individuals with ADHD

Many people with attention deficit hyperactivity disorder (ADHD) have been highly successful in their chosen fields. People with ADHD can take heart from these examples of perseverance and success. Some of the most well-known are as follows:

Sir Richard Branson: Sir Richard Branson, founder of the Virgin Group, has been candid about having attention deficit hyperactivity disorder. Despite difficulties in the classroom, he used his ingenuity and determination to found a multinational corporation that would change the world.

Simone Biles: Olympic gymnast Simone Biles has been open about her struggles with attention deficit hyperactivity disorder (ADHD) and how she uses her hyperactivity to her advantage in the gym. She has become one of the most successful gymnasts of all time, proving that people with ADHD can exhibit extraordinary levels of drive and focus.

Michael Phelps: Michael Phelps, Olympic swimming record holder, has been diagnosed with ADHD. He claims that swimming has helped him control his ADHD and improve his concentration. Phelps' extraordinary career and plethora of Olympic gold medals are the result of his hard work and dedication.

Solange Knowles: Solange Knowles, an actress and singer, has spoken candidly about her diagnosis with attention deficit hyperactivity disorder (ADHD) and how she has come to accept and even embrace her brain's wiring. She's established herself as a prominent artist in her own right, celebrated for her fresh perspective.

Justin Timberlake: Grammy-winning singer/songwriter/actor Justin Timberlake has been open about his struggles with attention deficit hyperactivity disorder. Timberlake is an excellent example of the adaptability and tenacity that characterize people with ADHD; he has achieved great success in a number of different fields, including music, acting, and business.

These examples of achievement show that having ADHD need not be a barrier to success. Instead, it puts the spotlight on the remarkable skills and strengths that people with ADHD often possess.

Inspiration and Motivation

Finding inspiration and motivation is essential for individuals with ADHD to overcome challenges and pursue their goals. Here are some ways to seek inspiration and stay motivated:

Role Models: Find people who have overcome adversity while managing their ADHD and model their behavior. Find out what they went through, what they did, and how they used their individual strengths to succeed.

Personal Reflection: Consider your own strengths and achievements. Recognizing and rewarding even the smallest acts of success can help you maintain a positive outlook and boost your self-assurance.

Supportive Communities: Participate in communities and groups for those with ADHD, where people can share their stories and offer encouragement to one another. When times are tough, it can be helpful to surround yourself with positive, supportive people.

Visualization and Goal Setting: Imagine the end result you want and make plans to get there. Create a plan of action, keep score, and enjoy small victories along the way. The ability to visualize success and establish concrete goals can be powerful sources of inspiration.

Self-Care: Focus on nurturing your mind and body by engaging in self-care practices that you enjoy. Taking care of your body, mind, and spirit increases your vitality, fortitude, and drive.

Mindfulness and Gratitude: Focus on nurturing your mind and body by engaging in self-care practices that you enjoy. Taking care of your body, mind, and spirit increases your vitality, fortitude, and drive.

CHAPTER NINE

Support and Resources

Seeking Professional Help

To better understand and control ADHD, it is essential to consult a trained professional. Here are some suggestions for where to find competent help:

Medical Professionals: Get in touch with medical experts in the field of ADHD diagnosis and treatment, such as psychiatrists, psychologists, or neurologists. Comprehensive evaluation, medication prescription, and symptom management advice are all services they can provide.

Therapists: Individuals with ADHD may benefit from therapy. Strategies and coping mechanisms to deal with ADHD can be provided by therapists trained in its treatment, such as cognitive-behavioral therapists. They are useful for learning to manage one's time and priorities, one's feelings, and one's confidence.

Coaches: Goal-setting, time-management, strategy-building, and maintaining accountability are all areas where an ADHD coach excels, and they are all areas where they help their clients tremendously. They offer one-on-one assistance in overcoming obstacles and reaching one's full potential in one's daily activities.

Educational Professionals: Children and students can benefit from the assistance they receive when they communicate effectively with their teachers and the school's support staff. Work together with classroom instructors, guidance counselors, and other special education service providers to arrange for needed modifications and assistance.

ADHD Support Groups and Communities

Joining a community or support group for people with ADHD is a great way to get the help, understanding, and resources you need. Here are some potential solutions:

Local Support Groups: Try finding a local support group that focuses on ADHD. In-person or online, these communities serve as a haven for people to connect with and support one another through shared experiences and perspectives.

Online Communities: ADHD-specific online support groups, message boards, and social media communities can be invaluable resources. Talking to others who have been down the ADHD road, asking them questions, and sharing your own experiences can help you gain perspective and make meaningful connections.

Parent Support Networks: Parents of children with ADHD may gain comfort and understanding by joining a parent support group. These groups provide parents with a place to go for support, information, and the chance to talk to others in their position.

Recommended Books and Websites

Numerous books and websites provide valuable information, strategies, and inspiration for individuals with ADHD and their loved ones.

Here are some recommended resources:

Books:

"Driven to Distraction" by Edward Hallowell and John Ratey

"Taking Charge of Adult ADHD" by Russell A. Barkley

"The ADHD Effect on Marriage" by Melissa Orlov and Edward Hallowell

"Smart but Stuck: Emotions in Teens and Adults with ADHD" by Thomas E. Brown

"You Mean I'm Not Lazy, Stupid, or Crazy?!: The Classic Self-Help Book for Adults with Attention Deficit Disorder" by Kate Kelly and Peggy Ramundo

Websites:

CHADD (Children and Adults with Attention-Deficit/Hyperactivity Disorder) - Provides information, resources, and support for individuals with ADHD: www.chadd.org

ADDitude Magazine - Offers articles, blogs, webinars, and expert advice on ADHD-related topics: www.additudemag.com

Understood - Provides resources and support for individuals with ADHD and learning differences: www.understood.org

ADDA (Attention Deficit Disorder Association) - Offers support groups, webinars, and resources for adults with ADHD: www.add.org

Individuals with ADHD and their support networks can benefit greatly from the insights, practical strategies, and increased understanding of ADHD that can be found in these materials.

Always consider a source's reliability and usefulness, and if you want expert guidance that's tailored to your specific situation, seek it out.

CONCLUSION

In conclusion, "The ADHD Advantage: Why Different Brains Thrive in a Distracted World" describes how those with ADHD have a unique perspective on the world and how they can take advantage of it. Throughout this study, we've considered the intricacies of attention deficit hyperactivity disorder (ADHD), the challenges experienced by those with ADHD, the distinctive features of the ADHD brain, and the strategies used to achieve success in a variety of contexts.

We have rejected conventional wisdom and adopted the concept of neurodiversity because we recognize that attention deficit hyperactivity disorder (ADHD) is not just a disorder but also a way of perceiving the world. Understanding the cognitive characteristics of ADHD has revealed that those who suffer from the disorder may be capable of highly original and unconventional lines of thought.

We have also looked into ways of improving executive functioning, creating a supportive atmosphere, and lessening the overall impact of ADHD on daily life. People with ADHD can benefit from these strategies in a number of ways, including enhanced concentration, higher productivity, more effective time management, and more overall success.

In addition, we have investigated how to flourish in today's distracting environment, discussing such topics as learning to ignore interruptions, increasing efficiency, and unlocking the untapped potential of those with attention deficit hyperactivity disorder (ADHD).

We hope that you will seek out professional assistance, connect with others who understand your experience with ADHD through a support group, and use the resources provided to learn more about managing your condition. These resources are useful for both those who have ADHD and their loved ones.

We concluded by celebrating those who, despite living with ADHD, have excelled in life and become inspirational figures. These examples show that having ADHD does not prevent one from achieving one's goals; rather, it highlights one's unique strengths and talents. A new perspective is encouraged in "Why People with ADHD

Succeed in a World of Distractions" by emphasizing the positives of ADHD rather than its negatives. It's a call to arms for the world to accept neurodiversity and value people with ADHD for what they bring to society.

If we can learn to recognize and cultivate the strengths of those with ADHD, we can help them succeed in a distracted world and make significant contributions to society. Let's collaborate on making the world a welcoming place for people of all abilities, including those with ADHD.

THE END